The IMPORTANCE of BEING LIFE LONG LEAN and STRONG

Robyn Reimers

Contents

Introduction

What Makes Me So Passionate When It Comes to Physical Fitness and Strength

This is how it all began.

With anything in life, there is always a good reason behind the things that drive us towards our goals. Call it life's purpose or simply the reason why we are put on the earth.

Here is a brief introduction that explains the reason why I left an occupation that involved working with technology to one of owning a health club. The bid for optimum health will always be the single most important goal in my life, as it has served me well from a very early age.

Although the last thirty-five years have been spent running and training at the gym, my journey actually began as a gifted maths-and-science student. Perhaps foolishly, I left school a lot earlier than I should have and followed my boyfriend at the time to the local technical college. Without giving a thought to where my life may head in terms of a career, I decided to sign up for a certificate of technology in electronics, which I completed a few years later.

During this period, which was early 1980s, factories were changing from pneumatics (control systems that use air) to the electronic types that are used today. Straight out of the college, I was immediately employed to support this change and assist with the implementation of these new electronic systems.

Keep in mind that this was the early eighties, when women did not enter these factories, let alone work alongside male colleagues who were fiercely opposed.

Although it is fair to say women do have it tough today, it pales in comparison to what I experienced working in industry back then—in particular, that time spent in the oil industry, which was union driven and male dominated.

At the time, when I first started my career, there was a strong belief amongst factory and industrial workers that women should not be allowed to work in industry and that they were a danger to themselves and others. They also used lack of strength and physical fitness as their main argument, with many of them willing to go to great lengths to prove this point, even going to such extremes as to place me in potentially life-threatening situations in a bid to emphasise their belief that women were dangerous in the workplace.

On day 1 in one such oil company, I was told by a fellow male colleague to perform a specific task, which was to simply remove a broken gauge. What he didn't mention was that the gauge was still live and active, being pressured by another backup pump in full operation and containing sulphuric acid of around 99 per cent at high pressure. If I hadn't been diligent—and let me tell you, I learned early on not to trust anyone—carrying out all the correct checks and simply doing as I was instructed to do, I would have ended up dead or seriously maimed for the rest of my life.

I needed a way to cope with this level of pressure and also the negativity I faced daily working in this type of environment, and this is where exercise comes into it. I used exercise as my coping mechanism and discovered that a healthy body also reflected a healthy mind.

Getting fit and strong didn't mean the bad wouldn't happen; it meant I could cope with it.

I immediately saw the benefits of physical attributes which assisted with stress relief, and a focus that wasn't going to undo me. I also felt that I could match them most times on the physical front, even doing better in areas where we had to climb to great heights.

The only thing I can honestly say that got me through this period of my life was being in the best health and shape of my life, as it provided me with the determination and resolve to keep walking into a factory of, say, 200 men, who I can blatantly say hated me, and cope with it. I had a mental toughness back then that is still serving me well today, and I'd love to give other young people or anyone I work with that same feeling.

My main purpose in life is to pass on what I know can really give you the edge in every area of your life.

If you honestly believe you don't have to be physically fit and strong to operate well mentally, then maybe, after you have read the following transcripts, you may think again.

Anyone who has to operate at a very high mental level will need to be physically fit.

To illustrate what I am saying, think about the women who have osteoporosis. When these women suffer a major fracture to their body, such as their hip, why is it that over 90 per cent of these otherwise healthy women actually die? Or take for example a male who undergoes major heart surgery; he has every chance of making a perfect recovery, but never does.

Health professionals can testify that physical trauma can often mentally undo a person to the point of no return and bring down their chance of recovery with it, even when they appear to have every reason to get well.

On the other hand, when someone gets a mental condition, such as dementia or Alzheimer's, when their brain function drops off, watch how quickly their physical body will follow suit.

Mind and body are interconnected, and both need to be in great shape. You might think you are performing well, but how well are you really doing compared to how well you could be doing if you were physically fit?

Getting people to operate well mentally and reduce stress all comes back to their physical health.

Up until recently, I had never had a major accident. It was only three months ago that I suffered an accident—a cyclist hit me at high speed when I was standing still. After suffering two major blows to the head (the second from when I hit my head as I fell backwards in an unconscious state on to the pavement), I am very lucky to be alive.

After a brain haemorrhage and three months of recovery, I am back into full training and completely unscathed. Although there was a degree of luck in that outcome, I am so glad that I am not standing here today wishing that I had of been a bit stronger before being knocked down. That would have been too late.

Fortunately, exercise and strength training have always been my drugs of choice.

It is amazing how some of the most confronting or painful periods of our life can be a blessing in disguise. As the saying goes, 'What doesn't kill you makes you stronger', although I always think that the order of that saying should be reversed into something like 'Getting yourself stronger will ensure that whatever you are facing in life doesn't kill you first'.

My lifelong passion has been everything to do with health and taking it to the next level.

Although I have tested and tried lots of programs in fitness and health, I have also benefited enormously from my previous working life, that being the work I did with control systems. Using my know-how in the area of control, along with some courses in physiology and anatomy, I have gained important insight into the way our body works with regard to preventing disease and improving health.

This book is a tool designed to bring the know-how of both aspects of my life together, using a lot of life experience and observation to hopefully change the lives of those who invest in it.

Come with me on a journey that will give you the know-how to get yourself into the best health and shape of your life.

Anti-ageing your mind and body is key to living the life you have dreamed about.

Anyone can do it if they follow some simple rules using a balanced approach.

Read on with the knowledge that change is about to happen when you decide the timing is right.

Make the decision now, and you will never look back!

Starting out doesn't have to be extreme
It simply requires movement and the time to think
With every step of intensity going forward
Capable of bettering the frame of mind

Chapter 1

The Mental Side Of Getting Into Better Health And Shape

When working with people, one thing has become very clear, they are usually only looking at exercise from an aesthetic point of view.

What we need to be all aware of is that the benefits of exercise and getting strong are not all about the parts that are visible from the outside. If your body gets healthier, your weight and size will always head in the right direction.

Unfortunately, CEOs and business owners are still of the belief that getting their employees in better health is all about reducing absenteeism when it is so much more powerful than that.

I truly believe that lack of self-worth or how someone feels about themselves is without a doubt the largest reason for lack of productivity within a workplace, as silly as that may sound.

Recently I worked with a couple of clients to prove this theory. I had them capture their thoughts and write them down on paper every two to three minutes for a day. Now I realise that this exercise in itself is totally unproductive, but it was extremely useful to both those individuals.

When we revisited their thought processes, it was almost an exercise in them beating themselves up for the entire day: 'Headache', 'Sore back', 'I am out of shape', 'Hungry', 'Shouldn't have had that coffee scroll' to mention a few.

These are perfect examples of how many times a day our subconscious or real beliefs come in to distract us from what we need to get done.

If those two women were in the best health and shape in their life, their ability to concentrate on the tasks they need to do in the workplace would be without this negative crosstalk.

We all know the feeling. Having a good feeling about where you are at, good energy, food sorted, the day just goes according to your plan. Your work improves 100 per cent, and you feel great about the contribution you make.

When you consider that the brain is in charge of every muscle contraction, is it any wonder that when we are mentally down or stressed, we aren't able to achieve any level of physical improvement.

Feeling motivated and in a great head space ensures that every minute of time spent exercising will be time well spent.

The Power of the Mind Is Needed in Exercise

Have you ever wondered why there are times when you leave your training sessions knowing you could have done more? Even when there is nothing physically holding you back, you just can't seem to cut it.

The answer could simply lie in the way that you think. With every muscle response being initiated by thought, desire, and need, it makes sense that the intensity with which we move our muscles will depend upon the intensity of our thoughts. If you are not motivated or are in doubt of your ability, it will be a bit like saying 'Stop' to your body when you really mean 'Go'.

So next time you hit your training session, make sure you hit it with purpose. Sessions of purpose mean better results. Better results will be all the motivation you need!

Remember that our brain is in control of our muscles and their ability to contract. If you are going to take the time to get to a session, make sure you hit it with purpose.

Body and Mind: A Lifelong Partnership

I have to admit that my recent head injury has made me aware of the role exercise plays in my life. Being physically out of action, I was strongly reminded of the vital connection between mind and body and just how much movement can change the way we feel.

I believe every one of us has a drug of choice, and mine is definitely one that relies on the exhilaration gained through exercise.

Whether we are mentally down or experiencing physical trauma, there is no way we can achieve optimum health until we get both areas of our life in order.

Physical trauma does have the ability to mentally undo the person to the point of no return, bringing down their chance of life with it.

A Step in the right direction is all the motivation you will need.

Although the mind and body need a strong connection, this chapter goes on to look at the type of thoughts that can interfere with achieving goals and moving forward.

Lack of motivation is usually a result of lack of success. It is so important to understand the right way to go about things, with great results becoming your motivation. The power of positive thought cannot be underestimated in any area of your life. It is impossible for good things to take place if our controller is not in the right space.

It is also my observation that the best results in weight loss have come about when a person comes into our club with the purpose of improving their health.

In these situations, they rarely consider their size at all, with this increased focus for better health being in proportion with the gravity of the situation they are facing.

The more dire the health issue, the more determined they are on the health improvements. The more determined they become in their quest for better health, the greater benefit they get in terms of shape. This gives further testament to the statement that weight loss improvements are delivered automatically when you achieve better physical health.

Moving more is a good way to get your head in the right space. Getting your head in the right space will take care of everything else!

Lack of Self-Worth Is a Huge Load to Carry!

Most people that embark on a weight loss plan or healthy-living programme are doing so with their body and health not where they would like it to be.

Clients of mine can often have a real internal battle going on when they are wanting to change their life but cannot seem to focus on the job at hand. This lack of focus and result highlights just how much energy and concentration is spent in the way they feel about themselves.

If we were to capture and take hold of every one of our thought processes at every minute of every day, then it would often be an exercise in beating ourselves up for the majority of it.

How you really feel about yourself will be with you twenty-four hours of every day. Not only does it take a massive amount of our energy and focus to self-loathe, but it directs all our talents, energy, and focus away from the things that are really important in our lives.

Age isn't a barrier to exercise, but the fact that you believe it is, is the real barrier!

Too Busy to Exercise?

Lack of time is the most common reason given by clients for not exercising. Although fitting in regular workouts when you are time poor can be a challenge, it is really simply a matter of choice and priority!

No exercise means accumulating calcium deposits in your joints through lack of use, losing your strength, and becoming a lot more susceptible to diseases. All the things in your life that are keeping you busy, such as your work and family life, balance delicately on your health and longevity.

Need to rethink your priorities? You bet you do!!

Frightened to Get Fit for Fear of Being Judged?

Always hiding at the back of each fitness class?

Being overweight or in a poor state of health is not something we can hide because people around us already know. Judgements are more likely to be cast on those that do nothing.

So if fear is standing in the way of better health, inspire onlookers by putting the attention back on yourself. The way you treat yourself will set the standard for others.

The goal for better health and real-life change will mean small steps forward in order to set them in concrete.

Are Your Friends Making You Fat?

Weight gain—is it contagious?

Do you ever find that you are more comfortable with putting on that extra five kilos when you best friend gains ten? Your peers, whether you realise it or not, are the biggest influence on your thoughts and actions.

Your level of comfort with where you are at will be directly related by those that surround you. Subconsciously, friends and peers can almost sabotage your chances of success for fear that you may be breaking away from the group and their ways.

The power of support cannot be underestimated, but your goals and the way you want to live need to be for you and not for the comfort of others.

Take charge of your life today, and surround yourself with people who are not only there for you in hard times but are happy to cheer you on in your successes.

Motivation

Motivation is the key to success. Without motivation, it is almost impossible to make moves towards better health.

Good results are the only thing that is really going to motivate someone to go on. My advice to anyone starting out is to take the first step towards bettering yourself and then to take the time to recognise your progress regardless of the magnitude.

It is difficult to feel positive if you don't see progress. Measure achievements in all areas and recognise what you have accomplished. If you got in an extra workout or two this week, pat yourself on the back for it, and see it as a step forward in recovery. If the scales or the tape move in the right direction, then know that you are headed for the body that you have imagined yourself in.

If the week did not go as planned, then look at where you can improve and understand that nobody has success each and every week. See your setbacks as opportunities, and use them to motivate you in a positive way, propelling you towards your goals.

Our bodies are capable of really great things
It is our minds that we need to convince!

Every Workout Counts!

Next time you are training, consider this.

Ask yourself some key questions: 'Is the training that I am undertaking really getting me to my goals, or is it merely killing time?' 'Do I really feel that I challenge my mind and body during each session?'

Effective training never needs to be questioned. You feel it instantly, and it brings much mental and physical release. It should be something that you look forward to doing rather than see as a chore.

Training with intensity and purpose is something anyone can do. Ability, goals, and distance covered may differ between individuals, but benefits gained do not.

So next time you hit a session, hit it with a purpose.

At least then you can walk away tired, but proud!

The Look of Determination!

Every now and then, I have to stop and think about how lucky I am to be in a job where I can make a difference to someone's health! When someone loses their health and well-being, their whole world can feel like it is crumbling down around them.

No matter how much money they have or how well they do in the workplace, these will not make up for the fact that their health and well-being are out of control. Even the most outwardly confident person can hold deep-seated negative beliefs when they aren't feeling healthy.

When working with someone who is starting out, there can be a moment in time when there is a real shift in their results. Something triggers them into a different mindset, and they really start to turn things around. This feeling rarely comes from a place where there is little or no result in the way they look or feel. Their new set of measurements or newly acquired skills become their motivation!

So if you are not feeling your best, get in and just get started! With a few good strategies and the right advice, you too may get that look of determination!

Getting the look isn't all about what others see from the outside; it is all about feeling it from the inside!

Six Weeks Out of Your Life or Six Weeks towards the Rest of Your Life?

Even though I love the camaraderie and interest that a weight loss challenge brings, it can have either a positive or negative result for the people in it. Although I am very much a fan of the show *The Biggest Loser*, that series is a classic example of this phenomenon.

When putting people through an intense program in a specific time frame, I am still very much aware that this scenario can either encourage someone to do their brilliant best or can inflict the sort of pressure that is detrimental to them in the long run.

Putting someone in the spotlight or in a competition can sometimes see them resort to a path that is short term, and this is completely detrimental to a sustainable outcome.

Putting a certain window or time frame on results will be fine for some, while it's an absolute deal-breaker for others. Pressure for some will be positive, while others will do much better without a specified time to achieve their outcomes.

So ask yourself a key question before signing up to your next challenge or programme—is it just six or twelve weeks out of your life, or is it six to twelve weeks towards the rest of your life?

Work Ethic and Getting Fit Are One and the Same!

Ever wondered why two similar clients with similar training backgrounds and abilities in equal training time frames can end up miles apart in their results?

It is certainly not a physical reason but often a case of work ethic. Work ethic in the training game is no different to work ethic shown at home or in the workplace. Those that have a good work ethic at home or at work bring that same dedication and planning into the gym.

It can also work in reverse. Those who manage to improve their health dramatically do develop a new way of getting around in the world.

Make the decision today to get started. Your body will thank you for it!

Getting a Healthy Dose of Endorphins Is Great for Our Mind

For a long time there has been much debate about whether or not there is such a thing as a runner's high. For those of us that get out there many times over, we already know that this is so, although the scientific world still struggles to measure it.

Endorphins produced by intense or prolonged exercise are felt by lots of the running population, with endorphins being chemically similar to morphine. This pain-relieving effect of endorphins is probably the reason that runners can be found to soldier on through enormous pain barriers, such as those found with stress fractures and other significant injuries.

So why is it that some people experience this high and others feel like they want to throw up?

It is thought that when the body is put under extreme load, the mind and body start to separate, with runner's high being experienced more so by long distance or intense sessions.

It almost only happens to those with a reasonable fitness level and also has something to do with a person's ability to tolerate pain or an individual's pain threshold.

One way to ensure that you reach this pleasant state is to ensure you warm up well. Launching into a run too quickly will almost certainly ruin the rest of the session. Runners that relax into the initial part of a run without pressure will see themselves enter this state at a point when their body starts to feel at ease and is ready to load up.

Some claim that the runner's high could almost be better than the big *O*.

Either way, warm up well, and just get out there and try it. Nature will deliver a healthy dose of endorphins to those that seek it.

Is Your Latest Injury Doing Your Head In?

We often think of an injury as being just a physical setback when it can have an even bigger impact on us mentally.

But did you know that an injury may just be a blessing in disguise? It is often nature's way of restoring balance back into the body and directing us to a new way of doing the things that we love.

The steps that we are forced to take with an injury will often give you a much better long-term outlook by doing things such as changing footwear, building new muscle groups, and changing routines. These are often the very things that are needed in the first place for you to achieve a personal best.

Elite athletes know the importance of a lay-off period, doing it annually to regenerate their body right down to the cellular level.

So if you are down and out with an injury, tell yourself you are happily going through a much needed period of regeneration, and you are going to come out of it with a whole new body and a whole new set of achievements as well. Your body will thank you for it!

Changing the Way You Feel Will Change Your Life!

The connection between your physical and mental health is one that we rarely think about, but put simply, you can never have great physical health if you are mentally down .

Improving mental function is not about improving your IQ. It is all about changing your self-esteem and your ability to motivate yourself to go forward.

Having a positive mental attitude is the key to changing our lives and our health for the better.

The Power of Support

Surround yourself with like-minded people who are striving for health and fitness goals. Reduce time spent with those that have a negative outlook on life. Provide support and encouragement to those around you, and it will come back to reward you tenfold.

Your Thoughts Dictate What You Become

Whatever we strive to achieve in our lives, we need to be focusing on a goal at the end in order to get there.

Visualising goals in life are the best way to drive you closer to them. Visualise the type of body and health that you want, then stay focused on this until you get there. Although it is referred to today as the law of attraction, it is really similar to some of the laws in physics. I do believe in magnetism and that thoughts and the way we feel about ourselves and our situations attract all the things that affect us in our life.

We always think that we will feel better about ourselves when we get into shape. Although this is true, we need to change the way we feel about ourselves first in order to achieve the better shape.

As we move on through this book, it will become perfectly clear that the mind is in charge of all physical improvements.

The goal for better health and real life change will mean small steps forward in order to set them in concrete.

If you are like many people I have worked with who are convinced that genetics are the reason you are overweight, I hope to convince you that learned behaviour is the reason you are where you are today.

If we were to take you out of your environment, then control everything you do, your chance of success would improve 100%. This is something I have been able to prove time and time again.

Weight Loss Is Not a Physical Challenge—It Is a Mental One

I have also discovered that people often have underlying or subconscious beliefs about genetics and their lack of ability to achieve real results based on them.

My observation over time is that genetics are not what makes one person's quest for health easier than someone else. Although certain illnesses are genetically inherited, a person's ability to push through or live with a condition is markedly different based on the way they choose to live. I really believe that learned behaviour is often the reason that body shapes and similar health issues are carried on from one family member to another. We only know one way to live, and that is the one we have learned growing up.

Having seen people transform themselves by changing the way they live is such a wonderful thing to witness. Genetics rarely ever play a part in a successful outcome.

If you think you can, you will!

Genetics Are Not the Difference between Success and Failure

I don't believe that genetics dictate success or failure. I believe that learned behaviour has a much bigger bearing on someone's life. You only learn by what you observe.

If you have ever sat on the sidelines at a local school's soccer match, you will no doubt have heard lots of comments about little Johnny or Harry being a natural sportsman. The statement is basically inferring that genes have everything to do with a sportsman or sportswoman's ability and that certain individuals are destined for success more than others.

An athlete's ability is probably only 20 per cent physical, with the other 80 per cent having to do with how they think and behave.

Might I suggest that it is probably the tens of thousands of hours of training and commitment that delivers success and being mentally motivated enough to do it. Having a parent whom you look up to as a role model is also a key driver in these young people, not the gene pool.

We can all become whatever we aspire to be.

Loving what you do and practising your chosen sport with a passion will more than take care of the physical skills. Physical skills can be taught through practice and guidance, but thoughts cannot!

If you think you can, you will!

Children will also model themselves on their parents' way of life.

Ask yourself, are you the best role model for your child when it comes to getting active?

If not, then there is no time like the present to make a start!

Chapter 1 In Summary

- Negative crosstalk can be with us many hours of the day. Improving our health will not only help us physically, it will benefit nearly every area of our life that requires a level of focus.

- Being in the right head space has nothing to do with your IQ and everything to do with how you feel.

- Learned behaviour makes us who we are today. Genetics rarely play a part in a successful outcome.

- Mind and body have a vital connection. With the brain in charge of every muscle contraction, is it any wonder that any level of mental decline can be physically destructive.

- Physical improvements will never take place unless you are in the right mental space.

- Too busy to exercise? Then consider that the very things that are making you busy balance delicately on your health

- Remember, there is no better motivator than a good measurement on the tape. Get in and just get started. Results will soon become your motivation!

- As a mental coping mechanism, exercise is second to none. Moving more will be key to improving your mental state. Make it your drug of choice!

- The power of support is a wonderful thing but your lifestyle and goals need to be for you and not for the comfort of others.

- We always think that we will feel better about ourselves when we get into shape. Although this is true, we need to change the way we feel about ourselves in order to achieve the better shape.

Chapter 2

Why You Can't Take a Shortcut When It Comes to Bettering Your Health

The real challenge for me in getting successful health outcomes for my clients is getting them to know exactly what it takes to achieve long-term success, and it does takes a certain time frame.

This is where my past working life with control systems and a bit of scientific know-how come back to serve me well. Speed of change in a measured variable will dictate how hard an opposing force will come back to correct the situation

Our bodies have sophisticated protection mechanisms that leave our technology world for dead. This is exactly why dieting can never work. Our body won't let any change come about that could otherwise spell danger.

Although dieting might be seen by us as a positive thing, your body may not see it in the same light. Unless it is actually improving our health, our body will ensure that balance is restored and will often overcorrect in the process.

Hopefully, the following paragraphs will give you some insight into transforming yourself over the long term rather than opting for a quick fix.

Why Is It That Our Bodies Never Let Us Starve or Die Holding Our Breath?

Your body won't let you starve just as it won't let you hold your breath!

Next time your child threatens to hold their breath in a bid to win an argument, rest assured that their body will protect them, with instinctive reflexes winning out every time.

Starving ourselves is a similar scenario.

We would certainly want our bodies to protect us from starvation if we got lost in the bush, so why on earth do we expect those protection mechanisms to not kick in when we starve ourselves deliberately in the form of a diet or periods of limited intake?

Protection by our bodies does not take into account whether starvation is positive or negative. It won't care that we want to look better in a bikini. It will simply see starvation as a measured variable that needs to be dealt with.

Once starvation has been measured, all control will be taken out of our hands, so stop starving, and start living!

The rebound effect of dieting will mean as much as ten to twenty kilograms on your body each time you go through such a cycle.

Sensible and clean eating, along with regular and consistent movement of your body, is the only way you will win out.

It may take longer, but it will come off and stay off!

Instant Gratification or Long-Term Vision?

When it comes to weight loss and improving health, nature has a way of making sure we go about it the right way.

The ability we have to resist temptation for an immediate reward will be the difference between success and failure when looking for results that are to last a lifetime.

If you liken this to the business world, smart companies are the ones that invest their time working towards a bigger picture rather than reacting impulsively to changes in their daily operation.

If successful long-term weight loss is your goal, then you need to set yourself a plan that involves and pans out over the long term.

Teaching your body to do well on nothing in the short term will see it do well on less than nothing at a later date. Reducing calories in week 1 will mean a further reduction needed at regular intervals in order to keep moving forward.

Setting a goal that is in keeping with the long term will increase the probability of you making real-life changes. Real-life changes are the ones that never see you going backward, taking your body to a whole new level.

The type of personality traits you hold determines your need for immediate reward. The person who is outgoing, ego driven, and lacks patience will have trouble setting a long-term plan. With the proper planning and guidance, these people can change their way of thinking.

So with all this in mind, put your ego aside, and plan an attack that sees you achieving your goal over the next twelve months and beyond.

Do it once and do it right, or battle it
out for the rest of your life.

Have You Thought about Your Goals and the Length of Time They Will Take?

The start of each year can see lots of us taking up the latest diet plan or health kick in a bid to undo some damage done over the holiday break. With so many programs out there on the market these days, it is really hard to know which one to choose.

So before you settle for that weight loss program or fitness fad, you may want to stop and really think about what is right for you and what will give you exactly what you need.

Firstly, you need to consider the reasons why you are overweight, and be really clear about exactly how long it took you to get there. Was it through lack of exercise, or does it have a lot to do with the emotional state you were in?

Once you answer these questions, ask yourself if the weight loss program you are about to embark on will fix these problems or not.

Chances are that your quick fix and calorie-deficient plan may only give you short-term weight loss. Although the weight loss will be great and may last a month or two, the real reasons behind your original weight gain will stay.

These important underlying factors will also be the reason why your weight will return.

So this time round, make your resolution all about doing things the right way.

Building the right mental and physical attributes while losing the weight will see you not only weigh less but will also *totally transform you* in the process.

Are You a Sprinter or a Stayer?

Getting into shape and improving one's state of mind can be likened to running a marathon.

Those that run hard at the start can often find themselves hitting the wall before they have hit the finish line. Losing weight and developing a new way of thinking is really no different.

If you have developed a negative mindset and managed to gain a lot of weight, I dare say that this did not happen overnight. So why is it that we think we can permanently undo this damage in just a few months?

Although twelve weeks can give you a great kick-start, with weight and size heading down, it isn't near enough time to develop permanent change.

Just like the tortoise running its race, improving the body in all its key areas and with a consistent approach will see the body put up minimal opposition, allowing you small but permanent moves in the right direction. If you end up like the hare, you will be great in the short term but will run out of puff soon after.

If your metabolism is already challenged, it is even more important that you go about things the right way. Getting fitter, stronger, and eating better will see you eventually win out. Short-term fixes that cannot be carried out forever will see you starting over back and even behind your starting point every time.

So stop being a sprinter, and start becoming a stayer.

Stayers may be a bit slower to take off, but they do get to where they are going in the end.

Just twelve weeks? Or twelve weeks towards the rest of your life?

Ever Wondered Why the Pounds You Lose Quickly Are So Hard to Keep Off?

Why is it that the five kilos you lost when you were sick fly back on with an extra five when you are well?

The answer lies in the way our body responds to large changes in what it sees as the norm.

The longer we sit at any given weight, the more the body will see this as normality.

Just because we desire or need to make a massive change from what we have been, it does not mean that the body will see it in a good light.

If you make massive reductions in your weight over a short period of time, the body will interpret this as a sign of ill health, setting off alarm bells to the brain.

Whether we like it or not, these distress signals will see the body pull out all the stops to increase our storage of fat and do it relentlessly until things come back into balance.

The fact that you attempt to resist the opposition it throws up makes it doubly effective, delivering a response that actually overshoots what is needed. This is where the extra five pounds comes from.

So be very aware that more is not better.

Nature has a way of ensuring we go about things in our life the right way.

Unless health markers are measured by your brain to be heading in the right direction, you will go into a battle that will see you lose each and every time.

Chipping away day after day will soon see you well on your way to achieving great weight loss today!

Real Beauty Comes from the Inside!

When it comes to looking healthy and feeling great, we all need some pampering from time to time.

The regular treatment from a health professional can definitely make us feel a lot better about ourselves. But having perfect skin and features isn't really what gives someone the edge with their looks.

If you look around at the sort of person that draws attention from others, it is usually those that have an energy about them and that healthy glow.

What we do to ourselves topically will always pale in comparison with the look that you achieve when you are healthy on the inside.

A powerful mind, healthy nutrition, and a strong body will make you realise the difference that real health can make.

Like most things in life, nature has a way of ensuring that we achieve goals in the proper manner. The only level of success that delivers a lasting result is where health is improved and the timing is right.

You don't have to be rich to be healthy.

You also don't have to resign yourself to lack of success as a result of your genes.

People who are willing to change do so each and every day.

''Consistency and Simplicity equal longevity''

Your Health Is Your Wealth

It is fair to say that health and wealth do not always go hand in hand.

Health is the one thing that puts us all on a level playing field.

It is the biggest leveller in our fast and modern world, with the very wealthy sometimes wining and dining themselves into an early grave.

People who are not wealthy need to consider that this is one area of their life where they could actually have an edge over their wealthier neighbours.

By being really smart about their spending and using their limited budget to practise clean eating and smart training, they may in fact be the envy of those who are deemed to be better off.

After all, your health is your wealth!

Chapter 2 In Summary

The most important thing to get out of this chapter is that when getting into health and shape, you need to be ready to do it over the long term.

Your body is a control system and control systems do not control well with spikes in their operation.

Excepting and controlling a process to a set-point is what I have looked at and analyzed most of my working life.

Every one of our bodily functions and health achievements depend upon control. I am yet to see improvements in any process that isn't moving at the right speed and going about it the right way.

- Sustainable and long term weight loss needs a speed of change that is deemed healthy. This allows the body to except the new set-point, allowing us to step forward with minimal opposition.

- Genetics rarely ever play a part in successful improvements in health and fitness. The people that surround you, along with the way you choose to live are everything to do with where you are currently at.

- Improvements in health and shape will only ever be permanent when done in a way that is as nature intends or the body assesses as achieving better health.

- Dieting, detoxing or anything resulting in loss of muscle mass spells danger to our brain. With loss of muscle mass taking away our physical ability to do things, any wonder it is high on the bodies priority of control. Once danger is measured, your goals will be met with an amplified and opposing reaction that is impossible to beat. This will be the reason you get further from your goals as the years roll on.

- Finally you need to ask yourself how many times you want to go through the 'weight loss challenge' or 'get fit for summer routine' I would like to think that 'once' is enough.

- Doing it once, means doing it right. Doing it right, means doing it for life!

Chapter 3

Great Nutrition Is the Key to Success

Whether your goal is improving what you look like on the outside or feeling fitter, healthier, and stronger, the nutrition that you take on is a common denominator and one that determines success.

When dealing with any new client, I always make sure that they realise the importance of nutrition in their quest towards goals.

Even when dealing with elite athletes, getting them to do the right thing outside the gym or off the sporting field will be the key to their success.

I also believe in making things easy—using a simple set of rules and a focus that improves their relationship with food rather than preparing them for battle, as is often found in other programmes.

When it comes to nutrition, unfortunately, many of you are still wasting valuable time on programs that simply don't work. Dieting doesn't work. Hopefully, by the time you have read this book, it will be like turning on a light switch. Just understanding some key concepts will make a difference in the way you go about getting your results from here on.

What would it feel like to have an eating plan where you don't have to go into battle with your nutrition and you don't have to count calories or weigh food, eating only when you are hungry? Well, there is such a plan.

Those that we label naturally thin are just not that focused on food. They don't put their emotions into it; they don't stress about it. They see it simply as a fuel, eating only when they are hungry.

In this nutrition section, we will look at asking some key questions, presenting some great facts, and taking on a simple set of rules that will allow you to make great choices without the worry or stress.

Busy people don't have the time to count calories and weigh food.

In my experience, delivering people some simple concepts can literally change their life.

For example, portion control can be as easy as people realising that the body will choose *quantity* based on *quality*. Hunger is the mechanism that makes us source food to deliver key nutrients to each and every cell.

If you take in food that is devoid of nutrients, then the hunger mechanism will stay on until the body gets all the nutrients it is looking for. If you deliver food high in nutrients, your body will be satisfied with what comes in and switch the hunger off. Designing menus using superfoods or maximising nutrients in your diet will have portion control covered without you even being aware.

The other important thing you need to understand is that when you are wishing to lose weight, you are really aiming to lose size.

When aiming to lose size, with fat cells taking up many times the space of muscle fibre, what you really need to do is lose fat cells. To lose fat cells, you also need to know that there is a specific way to go about doing just that.

Most people take up the challenge by restricting calories quickly and significantly into the body. When we do this, it is not the fat cells that are lost; it is the good part of your body's composition that is lost, your active tissue or muscle fibre.

For example, it is very hard to tell someone who has just lost five kgs in their first month of training that they are on the wrong track. This amount of weight almost certainly isn't fat, with the amount of weight in keeping with muscle loss. The fact that I also measure a mere 1 to 2 cms of reduction around their midsection, further backs up that their active tissue has been lost, being more compact than fat, which is certainly not a plus.

The problem with the above is that most of us are looking for the quick fix to a problem that stays with us 24hrs a day. What I can predict with certainty is that if we do not deliver a change in body composition that is better, then the amount of kilojoules used throughout the day will need to be reduced, making the period of success short lived and unsustainable. This means our plan is now undone, whether at this point the client acknowledges this or not.

If the example given above was a measurement of around 1kg of weight loss, along with 5 to 6 cms reduction around the waist, I would have been punching the air, even if the client was not. This is unfortunately a frustration that I deal with way too often. Hopefully as we go through the book, the light bulb will come on and assist to people to not measure success in line with the scales.

Your active tissue or muscle needs energy twenty-four hours a day just to hold itself upright and firm, so if you want to work out in your sleep, you need to build this active tissue and not do anything to lose it.

Fat cells can be likened to cockroaches. Starving them won't affect them. Not needing energy in order to survive, they lie around and therefore will last the distance.

The only way to consume these cells is to put our active tissue into a state of repair, and only then will these fat cells be consumed as a preferred source of fuel.

To succeed over the long term, you need to build a body that burns more calories rather than restrict calories in.

By dieting, you are killing your active tissue. You are killing your ability to metabolise fats and carbs in your system.

Reducing calories in week 1 will need a further reduction by around week 5 in order to move forward. The rebound effect of dieting can mean as much as an extra ten to twenty kilograms on your body each time you go through one of these cycles.

Let's start by simply looking at some concepts and messages that will get you to look at nutrition through a different set of eyes.

We will then consider five basic rules to get right so that you build a body that burns more calories rather than restrict calories into the body.

"Restrict calories into the body' or "build a body that burns more calories"?

Are You Eating to Live or Living to Eat?

Are you always counting calories and weighing food? If you are, then keep in mind that it is impossible to build a stronger, healthier body on a low-kilojoule diet plan.

Counting calories and weighing food puts all the focus in your life around food.

This unhealthy focus is the reason why most people have such a battle with their nutrition. Doing battle with food will ensure that the struggle goes on, with a lot of us simply giving in.

Having food weigh us down mentally takes away our energy to train effectively, kills our motivation, and lessens our enjoyment in life.

Eating clean, healthy food *in the right combination* will ensure your battle is over, leaving you energised, focused, and ready to take on anything!

Naturally Thin or Just Not That Focused on Food?

Do you have a friend that can't seem to put a foot wrong when it comes to staying in shape?

Those that we label as naturally skinny are often people that are not that focused on food. They don't put their emotions into it; they don't stress about it, eating only when they are hungry.

Going into battle with your nutrition takes enormous time and energy, leaving nothing to put into the areas of life that really matter.

So if your goal is to get in shape, free yourself from the scales and throw away those calorie counters. Put in a really great set of rules and then zero focus on food!

Eat clean, eat natural, and you will soon be well on your way to achieving your weight loss goals today!

Get your nutrition to where you want it,
then bring your body up to match it!

Don't Let a Big Weekend Do Your Head In!

Feeling guilty after that big weekend?

Clients often beat themselves up after a weekend of partying, fearing that all their efforts during the weekdays have been undone.

I tell them to simply put the weekend behind them and get back on the right road for the rest of the working week.

Remember, five steps forward with two steps backward is still forward!

Metabolism—How to Beat It!

Everyone differs in the time and ease at which their body responds to making improvements to health and reductions in size.

Let me also assure you that 99 per cent of the population have the ability to win out in the end without medical intervention.

There is real truth in the saying 'Rome wasn't built in a day'.

Sometimes the hardest-working clients achieve little or no result when starting out in a new healthy-living program.

You have to really feel for the individual that gets a poor measurement, particularly if they have been putting in a busting effort in their nutrition and training.

Even worse is the feeling they get from watching others doing the same program, really kicking goals from day 1.

The real difference lies in the individual and their metabolism.

My biggest fear for these challenged clients is that after month 1, they will revert to the easy path, adding a further burden to their already sluggish system.

If they were to stop and think about how long it has taken them to develop their metabolism, then is it any wonder that we can't undo it in the first month?

Every dieting program undertaken winds our metabolism back another notch.

It is all the more important that people with poor metabolisms don't teach their body to do well on nothing.

Anti-aging starts from the inside out:

Exercise benefits may be visible from the outside but never to the level to which they will benefit you on the inside.

Although age-related degeneration of our muscle mass is mostly seen in the inactive, the fact that it is seen occasionally in the active shows that there are other factors other than exercise that come into play.

Loss of muscle mass goes hand in hand with the loss of neurons or nerves responsible for every part of our function. Loss of nerves affect our balance and therefore ability to go forward.

So moving more each day will definitely put you in good stead, but unless you address every area of healthy living such as that of your nutrition, high blood sugars will play an even bigger role on your chance to succeed.

High blood sugars kill neurons that are giving you the ability to fire and contract muscles repeatedly. Diabetics are a classic example of this, with nerve damage the result of not keeping themselves in check.

Nutrition doesn't need to be complicated. It just needs to be what nature intended. Clean, natural food without additive is always a good place to start.

Going into battle with your nutrition can be a recipe for disaster. Don't weight it, don't count it, just know how to combine it and all will fall into place.

Simple, effective and ready to go solutions will make healthy living easy, without taking over your life.

Just get in and get started. Your body will thank you for it!

Yo-Yo Diets Are a No-No!

Our celebs are often a great example of the effect of yo-yo dieting and what it does to our bodies. Read on.

> The human body is undoubtedly the most intelligent of control systems.

> And just like any control system, changes to a measured quantity will generate an amplified opposing force to counteract this change.

> Therefore, losing size quickly will see the body pull out all stops to bring things back to a state of equilibrium, often overshooting in the process.

Lose size slowly, and your body will start to accept this new size as its desired set point with minimal opposition.

The message is clear. Chip away daily with clean and sustainable nutrition along with some regular movement, and you will soon be on your way to great weight loss today.

Active Tissue On or Active Tissue Off

It always amazes me why people are so delighted when they see large kilograms coming off the scales in a short space of time.

Large numbers off the scales means loss of the 'active' tissue that is metabolising fats and carbs in our system.

Your goal should be to change your body composition into one that has a lot more lean muscle and a lot less body fat!

Every bit of lean muscle you build will build an ability to metabolise fats and carbs in your system.

Every bit of lean muscle you lose will see you lose an ability to metabolise fats and carbs in your system.

Why Weighing Yourself Daily Is Not a Great Gauge of Success

Never measure your success with the scales!

If there is one thing I tell my clients not to do, it is to weigh in day after day.

One part of our body that gets seriously overlooked is one that can change our weight and size within a day. With over twice the amount of fluid than that of our blood system, is it any wonder that our lymphatic system can have a severe impact on not only our health but also our weight? It is one of the most important systems we have—cleaning up and detoxifying every aspect of our body.

Real metabolic changes don't happen overnight or even in a week. If our diet is full of acid, we are not sleeping well, or are experiencing a level of stress, this system can become sluggish and clogged, with an inability to drain.

Although cellulite and saddle bags can have a genetic link, they are also highly linked to a lymphatic system that is not flowing freely. An acid-based diet or a decent level of stress are usually the main culprits for this system to wind down.

Our blood has a pump, but this clean-up system for our body relies on muscle contraction to pump it in and around the whole network throughout the body. Activity is therefore essential for good lymphatic health.

I can testament to being centimetres smaller in the calves after just one good night's sleep, showing the difference that just one factor can have on measurements, not to mention weight gain.

So this week, tuck the scales under the counter, and try the following:

1. Work on getting better sleep quantity and quality.

2. Keep active with a good mixture of cardio and weights.

3. Keep stress to a minimum. Stress also produces acid in the body.

4. Eat lots of alkaline foods, particularly the reds, such as beets and cranberry (known to flush and detox the system).

Chapter 3 In Summary

- There will be no chance of long term success unless you achieve a body composition change for the better. ie: more muscle, less fat.

- Every bit of lean muscle you build will assist in your ability to metabolise fats and carbs in your system.

- Every bit of lean muscle you lose, will see you lose an ability to metabolise fats and carbs in your system.

- Restricting calories into the body will mean results will be short lived. Building a body that burns more calories means doing it once and keeping it for life.

- Restricting calories in week one will mean a further reduction needed by week five in order to move forward.

- The rebound effect of dieting can mean as much as 10 - 20 kg extra on your body each time you go through a cycle.

- Teach your body to do well on nothing, and it will do just that.

- Raised insulin levels will stop you from losing body fat. Stress, lack of sleep and poor diet are the key factors we can control here.

- Your body will choose quantity based on quality.

- By dieting you are killing your active tissue.

- Your active tissue works out 24 hrs a day just to hold itself upright and firm

- Fat cells take up many more times the room of muscle fiber. This is the part of our body we need to shift as it takes away from our health rather than assist it.

- Fat cells are unaffected by starvation. Liken them to cockroaches. They will last the distance!

Chapter 4

Nutrition: Five Simple Rules To Success

The following set of rules and concepts are a simple way to learn how to make better choices with regard to nutrition without the stress.

Your body is a sophisticated control system designed to take care of us at the cell level. Put simply, hunger is a mechanism for us to take in more food if the nutrients our body requires are not being met.

Our health and body weight will improve over time when we understand these key concepts essential for long-term outcomes:

a. Our body will choose quantity based on quality; high nutrients in food are the key to portion control.
b. Long-term weight loss will only take place in your body if your muscle-to-fat ratio improves for the better or is maintained at an optimum level.
c. Insulin levels must be controlled in order to lose fat cells.

A LIST OF THE FIVE RULES

RULE NO. 1 - EAT FOODS IN THER MOST NATURAL AND BASIC FORM

RULE NO. 2 - EAT SMALLER MEALS MORE FREQUENTLY THROUGHOUT THE DAY

RULE NO. 3 - HAVE SOME FORM OF PROTEIN AT EACH AND EVERY SMALL MEAL

RULE NO. 4 - INCLUDE A HEALTHY TYPE OF CARB AT EACH AND EVERY SMALL MEAL

RULE NO. 5 - IF IT ISN'T LIFE-LONG, THEN DON'T TAKE IT ON!

Rule No. 1 – Eat foods in their most natural and basic form—a natural form of portion control.

Rule No. 1 is all about eating foods as they are found in nature. Call it clean eating or eating like a caveman, this rule is really all about portion control.

You see, your body will always choose quantity based on quality. Taking in foods of a high nutrient level will see your body needing only small amounts to meet its needs.

Taking in foods like pasta—which is really just flour, filler, and water—will see your body looking for more in order to meet its needs.

Think about it. How many apples can you eat in a row? But when you modify these apples and make an apple pie, you can seriously do some damage. How about fillet steak and chicken breast? I reckon one is always enough, but when you look at modified meats (such as ham, bacon, and salami), we can really blow out.

So next time you sit down to a meal, ask yourself some key questions. Is the food you are about to eat straight out of the ground, off the tree, or a protein in its natural state? If it isn't, then find something that is.

Eat clean, eat natural, and you will soon be well on your way to achieving your health and weight loss goals today.

Rule No. 2 – Eat smaller meals more frequently throughout your day.

Rule No. 2 is all about eating smaller meals more frequently throughout your day. Now this is a rule that many of us break. Whether it is due to lack of time or lack of preparation, lots of us are guilty of having long and lengthy gaps between each sitting.

Now if your goal is to lose body fat and keep hunger at bay, then this rule is one you really need to get your head around.

Dips in blood sugar equate to hunger. Eating often keeps blood sugar steady, leaving you satisfied and with a lot more energy throughout your day. Now that doesn't mean eating for the sake of it. You should never eat more than you need. It is really all about splitting up your whole day's eating into smaller amounts.

Your body is really good at predicting future events. It also bases these future events on past behaviours. So if you have been giving your body small amounts often, your body will expect that pattern to continue.

Expectation of food appearing with frequency means the body will take the food in and put it to immediate use, knowing it will receive a hit soon after. If you have long and lengthy gaps between meals, your body will start to predict these gaps and start to prepare itself for them.

Long gaps between meals mean that food will be stored as fat for what it sees as a famine. Teaching your body to expect and utilise food coming in is the key to long-term success.

It is important to note that not all your meals need to be solid, so if you are really busy during your day or on the run, a liquid hit in the form of a smoothie or shake is a really great option.

Small meals give real benefit, so start giving your body small amounts often, and you will soon be well on your way to achieving great weight loss goals today.

Rule No. 3 – Have some form of protein at each and every small meal

Having some form of protein at each of your small meals is the key to losing fat, keeping insulin levels in control, and reducing hunger.

Building some muscle is a bit like growing a garden. Put in the right set of conditions, along with the proper training, and you will achieve your goals.

If I look at most of my clients' eating plans, I find that they are often eating really healthy food, but there is little or any protein earlier in the day, with them often taking in a large amount in their evening meal.

This is a bit like not drinking all day, then bucketing down a large quantity at the end of it in order to hydrate. It simply doesn't work!

Hunger seen in the evening often means there has been a deficit of adequate protein earlier in the day. At each of your small meals, make sure you have a small amount of protein in each and every one of them.

Knowing what you need and when you need it will be the key to your success.

Rule No. 4 – Include a healthy type of carb at each and every small meal

These days when we talk carbs, we straight away think of our starchy types in the forms of breads, cereals, rice, pasta, and potato. But not too many people think about fruits and vegetables as being carbs when, in actual fact, gram for gram, we can get just as much energy value from them. Not only are they great for energy levels, we also get lots of key nutrients from them, giving a massive boost to our health.

Without carbohydrate hits regularly throughout the day, you will end up tired, listless, irritable, and unable to think straight. Low-carb diets are a deal-breaker. They simply do not work. Every one of your meals should include some form of carbohydrate.

I like to split carbohydrates into two distinct categories:

1. starchy carbs
2. fruit/vegetable carbs.

As far as your muscles are concerned, there is really no difference in carbohydrate value between starchy foods to those found in fruit and vegetables. Sugars and starches may differ in their insulin response, but as far as energy goes, they both give sixteen calories of energy per teaspoon.

The real difference between the simple sugars found in fruits and vegetables versus the carbohydrate found in a starch has everything to do with their nutrient value and the impact on our health.

Fruits and vegetables are in their most natural and basic form; therefore, it is impossible to overeat on them. They give smashing health benefits, particularly if you choose those types that are dark and varied in colour. Eating lots of colour means a wide variety of nutrients and, therefore, improved health.

The real issue with our starchy carbs is that they are often accompanied by fillers and additives which can often react with our bodies, causing a rise in inflammatory conditions. They are also often bleached white, leaving them totally devoid of nutrients. No nutrients means the body will want a large quantity to satisfy its daily nutrient requirement.

While a lot of our starchy foods increase inflammation, fruit and vegetables are nearly all anti-inflammatory. With inflammation being the common denominator of all disease, eliminating these starches and replacing them with fruit and vegetables can make a massive difference to our lives.

So get your carb hit in its most healthy form—straight out of the ground or off a tree, just as nature intended. Do this, and you will soon be well on your way to achieving greater health today.

Preferred Carbs

Starches	Fruits	Vegetables
lentils	apples	asparagus
sweet potato	bananas	artichokes
black or wild rice	pears	avocado
steel-cut oats	plums	tomato
	nectarines	broccoli
	lemon/lime	cauliflower
	oranges	red/green capsicum
	grapefruit	onion
	berries	shallots
	watermelon	mushrooms
	pineapple	carrot
	peaches	celery
	black grapes	cucumber
	blueberries	lettuce varieties
	figs	spinach, kale, rocket
	pomegranates	green peas/beans
		snow peas
		eggplant
		chillies

Rule No. 5 – If it's not lifelong, then don't take it on!

Last, but not least, if it's not lifelong, then don't take it on. Rule No. 5 is all about getting long-term results. There are no quick fixes when it comes to sustainable and long-lasting results.

If your eating plan does not improve your health, then find an eating plan that does. If your eating plan is only good for ten weeks, then expect some sort of rebound once you return to normal eating.

Your nutrition needs to be lifelong.

Chapter 4 In Summary

- The five rules are put together to provide clean, natural food combinations that ensure insulin levels are kept in control

- If insulin levels are down and in control, body fat storage will be minimal.

- Taking out all the fillers and additives from our food ensure reactions and inflammation in our body is kept at an all time low.

- Combination and timing is so important in our diet. Building lean muscle is a bit like planting a garden. Putting the right nutrients in the soil and watering it at the right frequency will deliver maximum growth. So it goes for the training game. Eating small amounts often of food with high nutrient level is key to achieving your goals.

- Combining fruit and vegetable carbs with a small amount of protein at frequent intervals throughout the day is about as difficult as it needs to be.

- Simple effective rules can literally set you free and take your body to a whole new level.

Example of a typical day:

Breakfast: blueberry + natural A2 low fat yoghurt + one scoop of protein combined in a bowl, sprinkled with LSA

Mid morning: Boiled egg + vegetable sticks.

Lunch: Protein in a healthy salad / vegetable combo.

Mid afternoon: Black grapes + raw nuts

Dinner: Protein and vegetable / salad combo

Supper: Coconut / almond milk low fat combo with a small piece of dark chocolate.

Chapter 5

Train Smarter, Not Harder

Your body will be around a lot longer than that expensive handbag

Invest in yourself!

This chapter is all about ironing out some common misconceptions out there about the training game.

Training needs to be simple and consistent. It shouldn't be about smashing yourself but rather giving your body many different experiences, making it a well-rounded, well-thought-out approach.

It is important to note that weight loss success is not all about the type of training that is fast and hard. Reading through this chapter, some of the most effective exercise I can deliver clients with low fitness levels and a low strength base are in stark contrast to what moves them forward at a later date. Teaching a person's body to use fat as fuel is key in the early stages of training is something that a lot of other trainers do not see as useful.

Strength and *fitness* are attributes that you should *never* lose sight of.

Lots of people embark on a training regime to look better from the outside when as I have previously mentioned, it is so much more significant than that. It is really what's happening on the inside that is truly important.

Losing muscle fibre is really about losing functionality, which is all the more important as we age. If you liken our muscle fibres to an army, the heavier the load we lift or the more intensity with which we train, the more muscle fibres are recruited, and therefore the more muscle fibres are maintained each and every year. More muscle fibres giving more functionality means a better outlook for ageing. Let's face it; we all want to be able to do more as the years roll on.

Changing your body composition is seen as the best way of moving forward in a quest for optimal health, better function, and increased longevity.

The physical activities that we took on as a young person or teenager will have a significant bearing on the level of success that we achieve at a later date. Muscle fibres that have been built early on provide a base for further growth at a later date.

In saying that, it is never too late to make a change for the better. It simply means that you will need to work harder.

What worries me now about Generation Y and younger is the sedentary activities that make up their early years with the increased use of computers, phones, and games. We are now seeing the highest body fat levels to date from males or females, even in those between age twenty and thirty. Their bodies gain fat more readily without the underlying muscle fibres, unlike the young people in our generation that were active day after day.

Body composition is developed at an early age and is an important trait to pass on to our descendants and loved ones around us. It is the foundation that we build on in our later years and will have a significant impact on the level of result we can achieve at a later date.

Activity Is All Around Us

Mums are the ones out there doing us proud!

Although there is much talk these days about people becoming less active in our city, it certainly isn't apparent when out and about in the city streets and parklands.

You have only got to take a look at the increased numbers attending fun runs to know that certain groups are defying these trends.

Young mums, in particular, can be seen out there pounding the pavement, doing themselves and their families proud. When mum or dad gets fit, so does the whole family! Leading by example is the most powerful message you can deliver to those you care about the most.

Your health and that of your loved ones are your wealth! If you need a better reason, you will struggle to find one!

As you read on, you will see why some people do better than others when it comes to achieving success in the training game.

When I look for trainers to hire, I look for those with life experience. This isn't the type of stuff you can get out of textbooks. It is really all about observation and understanding what it is the client needs.

'We cannot do everything at once, but
we can do something at once.'

Crawl before You Walk, Walk before You Run, Run before You Jump

Whatever you are striving for in life, it will always involve completing a series of step changes in order to get you there. You need to master basic skills before you move on to more-complex ones.

Getting yourself in peak physical fitness is a classic example of where mastering fundamentals and building key attributes is an essential part of achieving success.

For example, if your end goal is to be able to bust out very intense sessions regularly of less than an hour due to your busy work schedule, then you need to have some basic skills under your belt to achieve it.

Endurance will be a basic attribute needed here, or you will simply bomb out of an intense session within a few minutes. Building endurance into your body requires you to undertake a series of steps that are actually in stark contrast to your end goal. An endurance build requires lengthy sessions of low intensity as a fundamental part of your plan, moving you through to the more-intense sessions as time progresses.

Understand and stick to your plan of attack. You will then be reaping one of life's greatest rewards—smashing health and fitness. Got to be happy with that!

Past Training History? Were You Athletic in Your Younger Years?

If the answer is yes, then you are going to do just great when it comes to getting back into shape.

A past training history can be likened to the early damage done by the sun, but in a positive way. Sun damage done in your younger years has a significant impact on you later in life. So it goes for the training game. The muscle fibres developed as a younger person will see you achieve a much firmer body well into ripe old age.

Mind you, it is never too late to start, and there's no better time to reignite those fibres than right now!

Use It or You Will Definitely Lose It!

We have all heard the saying 'Use it or lose it', but did you know that if you don't actively use your muscle fibres, you will lose them permanently to the ageing process?

If you think anti-ageing is all about getting your latest shot of botox, then think about the fact that you may wish to have a body that can live up to your new look.

Not only does exercise keep us firm, but the healthy glow that goes with it will definitely wipe years off your life.

Need a better reason to move more?

Five out of Seven Is What It Takes!

Setting goals is what the fitness game is all about.

Having your mind fixed on an end point is such a great way to make major achievements when it comes to weight loss and getting fit. Having a goal in mind is one thing, but knowing what it takes to get there is another!

If losing body fat is your goal, do not enter into it thinking that you will achieve great things being active a couple of times a week with your trainer.

When you are moving from one body type to another, the period of transition will be one that you really need to pull something out of the bag. I tell clients that they need to be active at least five days out of seven in order to move forward to their goals. Once they reach their end point, then they can maintain three or four sessions per week.

So set a task, rearrange your weekday schedule, and take yourself to a whole new level!

Life feels pretty great when you are at your peak!

Take Great Care of Yourself When Starting Out!

I always make a point of telling clients that are new to training that they need to ensure that they eat really well and get plenty of rest when starting out on a new training program. I tell them that they can liken themselves to that of a growing teen; long-lasting results require them to take on a whole new body composition.

Building this new body requires a huge energy load and sees quite marked hormonal changes in the process. Just like a teenager, this huge upheaval can make you quite susceptible to illness while this takes place.

Good news is, once you get a lot fitter and reach your goals, your immunity will get a much needed boost, making you a lot less susceptible and a formidable force in every area of your life.

Toned Muscles Are the Key to Working Out Twenty-Four Hours a Day!

During exercise, our muscles use energy to perform work. But once the workout finishes, so does a lot of the energy.

Toned muscles require a constant energy source to keep themselves firm, unlike flaccid muscle that is unable to support its own weight.

So even if your weight is not where you want it, keep on building your muscle tone. This is one way you will see your workouts extend to twenty-four hours a day.

Doing a workout in your sleep—gotta love that!

'Success does not come to you . . . you go to it!'

Pump Up the Volume for Maximum Fat Burning

More is definitely not better in the training game. Too much training or training of the wrong type and combination can be a real deal-breaker. Read on.

Teach Your Body to Use Fat as Fuel!

Ever wonder why those starting out in an exercise program struggle to lose body fat? If you believe that short, sharp sessions of maximum intensity are the only way to get results, then you may want to think again. People of a low level of fitness have very limited stores of carbohydrates in their muscles and liver. This ability increases with fitness, with elite athletes having maximum storage capability.

Low levels of fitness mean an unnecessarily high usage of carbohydrates. The energy supply from carbohydrates and fat are inversely related. The higher the rate of carbohydrates used, the lower the amount of fat used.

High rates of carbohydrates usage seen in the untrained person will mean that the combustion of fat will basically be switched off. Putting some 'volume' or length into our sessions is the only way we can begin to switch the usage of carbohydrates into targeting our fat stores instead.

Walk sessions or ones involving a light jog have intensity down low enough to stop the high usage of carbohydrate and, as a result, begin to teach the body to utilise fat more effectively and also increase our ability to store more carbohydrates in the muscles and liver.

Mix these longer sessions in with your short and sharp, and you will soon be needing that new wardrobe. That will be a good problem to have!

The Early Bird Gets the Results!

If you spend enough time at a health club, you will soon get to know that different times of the day attract different types of clients. Morning and afternoon users often have the same physical attributes, but their results can be literally miles apart when it comes to weight loss.

This observation has always fascinated me, with the morning group a standout winner overall. So why is it that these early birds really nail it when it comes to achieving their goals?

Here are a few good reasons why early risers do better!

1. Doing something good for yourself first thing in the morning makes you a lot more likely to eat well and do the right thing for the remainder of the day.

2. Morning training gives you that boost, firing up your metabolic rate for many hours after.

3. Morning training makes you feel positive from the get-go. Your mood can really impact on your ability to lose weight.

4. Although experts are divided on fuel theory, fuel usage may favour fat burning when the system is low in carbohydrates, such as that upon waking.

5. Morning training means your early session is a priority of your day. That trip to the supermarket or appointment will certainly not stand in the way of your 6 a.m. session.

6. You will be more likely to sleep better and go to bed earlier if you are working out in the morning. Every hour at the end of the day you stay up can mean that you may need to stay in bed longer to get the equivalent sleep needed in the morning due to the light after dawn. Bad sleep patterns are also a deal-breaker, making it almost impossible to shed kilos.

Still no good in the mornings? Then maybe it's time to change!

Warm Up Well until You Feel Your Second Wind!

If you have ever gone out too hard at the start of your training session or in a fun run, you will probably find that you will have hit the wall pretty soon after.

Lots of people neglect their warm-up, thinking that they will be saving their energy for the best yet to come. Nothing could be further from the truth! Not bringing your body gradually up to speed in your run session is a bit like hitting heavy weights at the gym without any sort of a warm-up.

Your heart and cardiovascular system can be likened to any other muscle or joint in your body. Loading up without preparation can be damaging, with the body forced to pull out all the stops to protect itself when this occurs.

Whatever your fitness level, running flat out from the get-go will force the heart and its arteries to dilate at an exaggerated rate, winding the heart up to dangerous levels to do so. The body detects a dangerous situation developing and will start to douse your muscles in lactic acid. It will also start pulling enormous amounts of carbohydrates out of your system at the very same time. Once your muscles are doused in lactic acid, you will not do well for the rest of that session.

These protection mechanisms are a good thing. Imagine if we didn't have an inbuilt limit. We would simply overrun our heart, damaging ourselves permanently.

The smart way to run is to start off slow or spend twenty minutes prior to your event bringing your body up to speed, with a few run-throughs towards the end of this time. Once you are comfortable, you should then stop and reset yourself.

Start slow, reset, and then take yourself to a new level!

Free Weights vs Machines—Both Have Their Place!

There are so many new trainers coming on to the fitness scene with the belief that machine-based leg exercises are a waste of time and only for those that want an easy out! Nothing could be further from the truth!

Without a doubt, free-weight moves—such as the squat and dead lift—are simply some of the best moves to build your body. However, they also demand a high degree of accuracy in their execution to avoid serious injury.

Over the last thirty-five years, I have witnessed lots of bad technique and resulting injury in the process, with even the experienced bodybuilder sometimes coming undone when they have gone up into very heavy weight sets.

Other factors to consider when looking at your client base is that around age forty, physiological changes happen that make tissues and supporting structures more susceptible to injury. For example, age sees meniscus hardening in knees, which presents risks if execution of moves is not flawless.

With a large percentage of my clients in the forty-plus age group, I like to see them in a safe and set position, really loading each muscle group up first before progressing them into the free-weight moves and then doing so at a lighter weight set.

Athletes that do triathlon and similar sports exhibit power-to-weight ratios that would challenge most others. They are right into the machine-based weights with higher rep ranges but pushing around two and a half times their body weight with single legs. They also practise balance and functionality with free weights but again at a lighter weight set.

Whatever tool or move you use at the gym, make sure you do it safely. Your body will thank you for it!

Weight Gain Is a Vicious Cycle!

Did you know that weight gain and painful inflammatory conditions go hand in hand? Those that carry the most weight also carry the biggest burden when it comes to painful conditions. Painful conditions such as arthritis are exacerbated by an increase in weight. This pain often makes it very hard for the larger person to want to get active, let alone train day after day!

Even though it may be painful to push through at the start, chipping away with a well-rounded approach to your whole lifestyle will see you eventually win out. Some amazing life-changing transformations are testament to the fact that this cycle of pain and frustration can be beaten.

Breaking the cycle means consistently chipping away in all the key areas of lifestyle rather than trying to take a flying leap in one direction only. Persistence is the key. Moving the right way and getting your body in good health will be the strongest anti-inflammatory you will find!

Muscles Need to Be Strong in Order to Switch Them On!

When someone is starting out in the weight training game, it is often a real catch-22. The client new to weight training needs to focus on strengthening specific muscles and often those that prevent injury around their major joints.

In order to train these smaller assisting muscles, it requires them to be switched on effectively from the brain. Unfortunately, being able to fire these muscles neurologically is much more difficult when they are weak.

So if you are starting out in the weight training game, take it easy at the start. Rome wasn't built in a day. Some lighter weight sets with a bit of key focus is the key to moving to that next level. Those that get the balance right end up with muscles that can be activated on time and every time they are needed.

Strength and focus will be the key to your long-term success!

Increasing Endurance

Building endurance requires our muscles to store carbohydrates more efficiently. Carbohydrates we eat are converted to glycogen, and are stored in our muscles and liver.

You can liken the storing of fuel in our muscles to that of energy stored in a battery. To make a battery more efficient at storing charge, it is often best to discharge it fully. Similarly, our muscles become better at storing fuel with increased training, particularly the long slow-distance type that sees us deplete these stores significantly.

Training to a point where muscle fuel reserves are significantly depleted will see the body adapt with a bigger reserve in weeks to follow. Aim to increase volume of your training by around 10–15 per cent each week to achieve maximum efficiency. Maximum efficiency means easy running at a time equal to your personal best.

Take a Well-Rounded Approach to Your Training!

With so many training options available today, it is really hard for people to decide which one to choose. Whatever road you decide to take will hopefully build a certain set of attributes needed for all-round health.

Fitness is one thing, and strength is another. Often choosing just one type of training option will see one of these key attributes sacrificed in favour of the other.

If running outdoors is your thing, then do not underestimate the benefit to this beloved activity that a regular session at the gym may bring. A strong cardiovascular system is not going to be able to cut it if it has to drag a weak set of muscles or core along with it.

A strong structure is a key attribute needed for longevity, and training must be specific in order to achieve the right result. By all means, sign up for the latest fitness craze or run group, but for the price of a few cups of coffee, consider the extra spend that will give you real longevity.

Your local gym is a superior environment in which to get your body strong. Weather is never an issue, and every different ability level can be catered for. A gym or a health club can provide a wide range of safe and traditional moves needed to give real strength in the shortest possible time frame.

So if you are looking for a total health solution, don't ditch one training option for another. Good food, effective and well-rounded training, and the power of support are things that you should never be without.

Look Beyond the Sight of Injury!

Have you ever wondered why our joints are not all made by similar design? Understanding the intention of this design is the key to remaining injury-free. If you look at the body's major joints, you will see that these points of movement in our body alternate between stabilisers and mobilisers.

Mobilisers are the joints that give us a larger degree of movement and are the ball joints, such as in the ankle, hip, and shoulder. Stabilising joints slot in between the mobilisers and are more limited in their movement. These joints are those in your knee and those that support the spine.

To keep our body functioning properly, we need to understand the importance of keeping the mobilising joints mobile and the stabilising joints stable. If a mobilising joint is restricted in movement, the stabilising joint next in line will need to move outside its preferred plane of movement, with a degree of injury to follow.

A sore lower back may have been caused by a hip that doesn't move well, with the lower back trying to rotate in compensation. Sore knees may be caused by lack of movement in ankles or hips.

So if your body feels out of whack, my simple solution is to focus on strengthening your stabilisers and stretching your mobilisers.

Sounds simple? Absolutely—it is!

Core Training—Not Just about Looking Good in a Bikini!

Most of us are told at some stage to strengthen our core, but how many of us understand what it really is?

Think of your core as a natural corset or tight bodysuit designed to hold in our most important body parts. Now imagine tightening that corset and the effect it would have on the way you look and feel.

Abs are the muscles that are visible from the front. To get these muscles strong, we actually have to provide them with a firm base. This firm base belongs to our core, and it encompasses an entire area designed to support the spine and central nervous system.

Core muscles include muscles in the front, back, and sides of our trunk, as well as those in our back and also our glutes.

If getting fitter is your goal, your core is connected directly to your diaphragm. Improving core strength will actually increase your lung capacity. If balance and coordination is something you would like to have more of, then your core is the centre of your universe and needs to be in good health.

Is core training just a fancy word for toning abs? Not likely!

Don't just build abs to look good,
they are vital to your stride!

Chapter 5 - Train Smarter, Not Harder: In Summary

- When starting out with your training, aim for five active days out of seven. Not all of these sessions need to be fast and hard. Two to three training sessions building strength and fitness combined with two active recovery sessions in the form of a walk, would be an ideal place to start.

- Getting yourself into peak physical fitness requires you to master the fundamentals and build the right base.

- Aim to do the type of training each week that recruits the maximum amount of muscle fibers. Give yourself a well rounded routine that loads you up doing moves that involve the whole body. The more muscle fibers recruited, the bigger the calorie burn. This will ensure you lose a minimal amount to the aging process. Recruiting more will see you lose less!

- Your past training history will come back to serve you well! It plays a significant part in your ability to achieve at a later date.

- Putting your training in at the start of the day is one of the best ways to achieve your goals. Nothing gets in the way of it and the mental benefits will carry on for the rest of your day.

- Getting muscles strong is necessary for us to be able to mentally switch them on. Just get in and get started.

Chapter 6

Tips For Runners

Training for That Next Marathon?

Sometimes you have to go backwards in order to move forward!

Putting in the hard yards, but still can't go the distance? Getting out of puff every time you hit the hour mark? Maybe it's a simple case of your body not having the right base!

If you have to be going at a fast and furious pace in all your training sessions, then chances are, your muscles will contain a lot of fast-twitch fibre. These fibres allow you to deliver explosive contractions to your muscles and are the key to being fit and strong. Trouble is, these fibres are not fatigue resistant and do not go the distance!

We all genetically inherit a combination of both fast- and slow-twitch fibres, with some people inheriting more of one type than another. There are also a good bunch of fibres that can be converted or could swing either way depending on the way you train. They can sway towards speed and power or that of the type that has endurance, and are resistant to fatigue. It is the latter of these groups that are needed in a marathon or long-distance event.

If you continue to always train at a fast pace, all your convertible fibre will swing towards fast twitch, and the distance you will be suited to will be more like 400 metres rather than a marathon. Hence, this is the reason you never see trained sprinters running marathons. They just don't have what it takes.

Taking a step back and training initially at a very low heart rate for increasing amounts of time each week will see you build more slow-twitch fibre in your muscles. These fibres will in turn be the very reason you will be able to run faster and longer at the same level of exertion in the weeks leading up to your event. Faster, longer, and at a lower heart rate will soon see you well on your way to getting that hard-earned PB.

All fast and hard will never see you tackling a marathon. Take the time needed to get your base right, and that marathon will soon be able to be ticked off your bucket list.

Running and Weight Training—A Formidable Force When It Comes to Weight Loss!

A lot of our clients, particularly women, are convinced that they were never meant or are never going to be able to run. This is such a shame, as running is the best way for us to get our clients to their goal weight. Running is one of the few exercises that use every muscle fibre in our body to perform each action. It also is an exercise where you are bearing your own weight, unlike exercising on a bike, rower, x-trainer, or pool, which sees your weight supported. It is also a quick and cost-effective way to train.

Running on its own can be very taxing on the body, but throw some good strength and conditioning into the mix, such as a few good weight training sessions, and we have the ultimate fat-burning programme—a formidable force against weight and size gain!

Strong joints and muscles make the act of running a breeze! It also ensures that you will run well into your sixties and seventies! Neglecting strength and conditioning routines will see your running career come to an early retirement!

Women need to strap themselves in, wearing two crop tops or sports bras to avoid the discomfort of breasts bounce. They also need to be given the right resistance training routine, one that is progressive and specific to achieve better running technique and form. The right routine will assist their muscular endurance and should be similar to that used by triathletes and runners to give a leaner look as well.

In my opinion, the gym is still a superior place in which to weight-train, particularly under the watchful eye of a trainer.

Balance and Symmetry—More Than Just Running a Straight Line!

An injury to your body is a quick reminder to all of us that something is out of balance. More of us than ever are out there pounding the pavement in a bid to de-stress, get fit, and keep unwanted kilos at bay! Every now and then, our bodies remind us that this beloved activity is in need of a more balanced approach, with injury appearing on one side of our body.

So why is it that runners will continue to battle with these imbalances and push through enormous pain barriers? The answer is simple—they love it too much to give it up!

Getting back on your feet after an injury to the body will mean change.

Sometimes we have to take a step backwards in order to go forward. The long-term benefits that will come as a result of this new direction will not only see you back out on the road to recovery, but it will be the key to taking yourself to a whole new level.

Running a straight and balanced line can wipe off many metres in your next fun run as well as keep you from having to hang your shoes up for many weeks on end.

Here are my tips for putting the balance back:

1. Get off the road and on to the treadmill—at least a few times per week. Treadmill running may not see you activating your hamstrings as much, but it will soften the blow under your feet while your body repairs. It will also ensure that you build much needed core strength, as you are forced to switch it on repeatedly or lose balance while running on the moving belt. Moving also within the confines of the moving belt will make you a tidier, more balanced runner when you get back out on the road.

2. Get back to the gym. Strength training using a unilateral approach (single legs) will see you loading up weak muscle groups in a controlled environment. Doing extra sets and repetition on your weak side will produce even strength and even usage of both sides of your body in the space of just a few weeks.

3. Use your downtime as a much needed chance to build on your endurance base. Longer low-intensity sessions will see you building on your slow-twitch fibre base, giving you the necessary platform to run harder, longer, and faster when you are back to your peak.

Better strength on both sides of your body means two powerful legs instead of just one!

Changing Your Body Type Could Be as Easy as Changing Your Shoes!

Ever put on a new pair of runners only to find you are terribly sore all over the first time you run in them? The fact that your muscles are sore often means that you have recruited extra muscles or challenged them in some way.

Heavy footwear means our muscles in our legs and feet will not have to work as hard. Light shoes require a lot more of our bodies, recruiting a lot more assistance from muscles that will otherwise lie dormant. More muscles recruited means more speed and power when you need it!

Remember, Rome wasn't built in a day. But going a few grades lighter will see your body get a lot stronger!

Strong body equals a healthy life!

Training for a Stronger, Healthier Heart

If you are running nicely over distance but struggling to improve your speed and run times, you may need to look at upping the intensity in some of your training sessions.

Although endurance is really important, the heart is like any other muscle in your body. To make it stronger, you need to put it under some sort of load.

Working at a higher rate, even if it is for a shorter time, will be just what you need to develop a healthier and stronger heart. With a great base level of endurance, going that extra bit harder a few times a week will not only increase your fitness but will burn calories for many hours afterwards, with the after-burn effect similar to that of weight training.

Love Running? How Long Do You Want to Run for?

Lots of people love to run. There is no better way to recruit all your muscle fibres, keep unwanted size at bay, and get yourself into the right headspace for the day. But how many of you are taking the correct steps towards being able to continue this great activity over the long haul?

Dragging weak muscles along means that your heart and lungs have to work doubly hard. Weak muscles also mean that you will be placing much greater load on all your joints as you go forward.

Injuries are so frustrating but can sometimes be so easily avoided. So if you want to run your personal best or simply run well into old age, ensure that you get the right strength and conditioning under the watchful eye of a great trainer.

Your body will thank you for it!

Strength—The Key to Making Good Runners Great!

Running is undeniably one of the most time-effective forms of training.

Those of us that are out there pounding the pavement or hitting the treadmill already know the mental benefits that come from this type of activity. Working every muscle fibre simultaneously ensures that we are targeting our fat stores and increasing our fitness within the shortest possible time frame. We also know how quickly we can regress once we are injured and out of action.

So why is it that most of us launch into this activity with little preparation or strength? Running without doing the appropriate strength training is like building a house without the right foundation. Strong muscles with the ability to fire repeatedly will give your heart and lungs the helping hand they need, making your run session a breeze.

Your local gym is definitely a superior place to get your base built, so what are you waiting for?

Runners Don't Build Abs Just to Look Good—These Are Vital to Their Stride!

Did you realise that your core and abs are the key to your success as a runner? In fact, they are the key to the power, speed, and endurance in your legs. Marathon runners will often fail in their core before their legs give out.

Building abs is not about doing endless sit-ups and crunches; it is about activating the right muscles and is often trained using an upright position. Your core should be a key weekly focus of your training right from the get-go!

A strong spine, powerful legs, and the ability to hold yourself very upright as you run will get you a PB without even raising a sweat!

Think the Treadmill Is a 'Soft' Runner's Option? Then Think Again!

What is better—treadmill or out on the road? It is really a matter of choice, but here are the pros and cons of the treadmill.

Advantages

- Running on a treadmill ensures that you are continually switching on your core in order to run within the confines of the moving belt. The faster you run on it, the more your core will have to switch on to stay balanced.
- Running on a treadmill often sees you running in a really tidy manner due to the confines of the moving belt. Most runners tend to take this balanced approach with them out on the road.
- The treadmill has less impact than the roadway. This is great for those that are doing long miles or are new to running.
- The treadmill allows you to set a programme and measure your results with ease.
- Not weather dependent.

Disadvantages

- A treadmill, with its forward-moving belt, promotes the type of gait that has limited hamstring activation. This can cause problems with the knees if not balanced with the right training or some road running.
- Road running has a degree of difficulty equal to a 1 per cent incline on the treadmill. More energy therefore is used on the road per minute of activity and therefore a better calorie burn.
- Treadmill running can be dead boring. An iPod is required.
- Treadmills can malfunction. Great videos on YouTube are a testament to this!

Whatever road (or belt) you take, keep on running. Your body will thank you for it!

Chapter 6 In Summary

- Running without the correct strength base is like building a house without any foundation

- Changing your footwear up will ensure that your muscles in your legs and feet don't suffer from overuse.

- Changing footwear means recruiting a lot of muscles in our feet that would otherwise lie dormant. More muscles available means more stability. More stability means less zig zag and less energy used out there on the run.

- Marathon runners often fail in their core before their legs. Core strength is not about looking great in a bikini or having a six pack, it is vital to your stride.

- Training for running should be specific to the event or goal your are working towards. Sometimes we need to take a step backwards in order to go forward.

- Running technique is not just about winning races, and more about not having to hang your shoes up early due to the body breaking down. I like to use the analogy in running similar to what cyclists use when looking at improving each stroke of their pedal. Developing your stride to where it sees the feet pulling the ground underneath you rather than throwing all the energy downwards into the ground is a good place to start. Run smarter, not harder is the message here.

Beating Bones Up Only Makes Them Stronger!

Did you know that every time you set out on a run, you are actually inflicting some damage to your bones? But not all damage is bad! This so-called damage is the very reason that you end up with nice, strong bones to support you well into old age.

The micro-fractures that appear in our bones due to running tell the body that they are injured and need to be repaired. The repair process involves building bone around these micro-fractures, with the same bones coming back bigger and stronger than before, ready for the next round of activity.

Beware, as more is not always better. To build a stronger skeleton, these runs need to incorporate the right rest periods to ensure these fractures don't exceed the repair. A few rest days a week are usually adequate to achieve the right result.

So do your bones a favour, and start hitting the nearest pavement.

Your body will end up thanking you for it!

Chapter 7

Pre- and Post-Workout Guidelines

Getting great results often means training well into a fat-burning zone. If clients, particularly those new to training, do not ingest some carbohydrate pre the session, they will struggle to hit this important zone with their body only consuming carbohydrates throughout.

Pre-workout Nutrition Guidelines for Optimum Performance

Food consumed before exercising is only useful once it has been digested and absorbed; therefore, you need to take in the right food at the right timing before training or your event.

Prior to training sessions that involve cardio—such as running, cycling, or swimming—your body will need carbohydrate as its main source of fuel. People often load up on lots of protein or foods high on fat, which can actually work against you when out there on the run.

> Ninety Minutes or More before the Session
>
> - oats or crumpets.
>
> Thirty to Ninety Minutes before the Session
>
> - banana
> - fruit smoothie.
>
> Inside Thirty Minutes
>
> - sports gel
> - sports water
> - rehydration formula with adequate carbs.

Fuel up Well before Your Workout—100 Calories Could Make All the Difference!

The biggest battle I have with my clients, and particularly my running groups, is getting them to see the benefit of adding some calories to their pre-workout nutrition. This is the one time that I recommend they take in a good hit of sustainable carbohydrates in the quest for maximum results.

No matter what your fitness level is, you do not want to limit a session based on the carbohydrate storage capacity of your body. The untrained individual has minimal storage capacity. Athletes and those at the higher level have a great ability to store carbohydrates in their muscles and liver. They also would never skimp on this area of their pre-training preparation.

Most clients with limited fitness ability will therefore only be able to sustain around thirty minutes of effective training, even at lower intensity, without taking in the proper nutrition. If at any time during that thirty minutes, they experience a high heart rate, they will probably chew through the remaining storage in around two minutes.

However, if those same people took in the extra 100 calories in the form of a sports gel, I have observed that these same clients are able to put in around two to three times the volume and sustain a much higher intensity of training as a result, with sometimes burning around 500 calories extra in the session. They are also able to hit a fat-burning zone during and after where there is an after-burn effect due to the higher intensity of the session.

So the question is, should you add 100 calories to achieve an extra 500 while also burning fat for many hours afterwards, or should you bomb out in around thirty minutes, failing to achieve greater goals?

You do the math!

Post Workout for Maximum Recovery—

Do You Want to Be Able to Train Harder, Longer, and without Injury?

Ever wondered how our Olympic athletes are able to bounce back into their hard training day after day?

Backing up training sessions with great recovery is the key to the reason that they are at the elite level of their chosen sport. The success in their recovery will almost certainly depend on what they take in post training.

Speed of delivery is the most important factor when it comes to refuelling well. Your post-workout nutrition should be almost the opposite of what is normally prescribed for healthy eating.

While normally recommending that clients eat slower-digestible carbs and slow-release proteins throughout the day, post workout it is important that they ingest carbohydrates that are high GI, with fast-release proteins, preferably in the liquid form.

Fresh-squeezed juices post training will ensure your antioxidant levels and carbohydrate stores in your liver and muscles are topped back up. Follow it up with a scoop of protein and natural yogurt with your breakfast, and you will be on your way to bigger and better things.

Being able to train with greater intensity more often without injury means greater body fat loss overall.

Great recovery gives great gains!

Juicing for Recovery

For those of us who like to train hard or back up our training sessions daily, there is simply no better way to replenish tired muscles than taking in a fresh fruit/vegetable juice.

Backing up day after day, such as that done by someone in a twelve-week program or in training for an event, means that you are putting your body under load on a regular basis. Most of us think it is better to eat your fruit and vegetables rather than take them in a liquid form. For most of the day, this is true, but when it comes to post-workout nutrition, speed of delivery is everything.

Taking in a large array of nutrients in liquid form straight after training ensures maximum recovery, allowing you to bound into your next session. Think of what works best when people are in a poor state of health. Often a juice hits the spot without the added load of digestion.

Know what and when it is needed is key to success.

Too Tired to Put Out?

Maybe you didn't fuel up before your workout!

Achieving goals means putting in cracking sessions where you walk away tired, but proud. Saving calories during these times is counterproductive. You will bomb out long before you have achieved your aim!

Your body needs carbohydrates for training, particularly if we are talking about intense cardio routines or running sessions.

Leave your protein hit until after training, as it is great for your recovery.

Chapter 8

Hydration: A Fine Line

Hydration is always an interesting topic, particularly in the training game.

Here are some tips that will make you think about how much of this vital fluid you should take in for optimum health and improved performance.

Water—Are You Drowning in It?

These days there is plenty of info out there telling us to drink more water. Lots of us are guilty of not taking in enough of this vital fluid. But did you know that it is actually possible to literally drown in the stuff?

We now know that most of the people that died on the Kokoda Trail fell victim to this illness, drinking relentlessly to replace sweat from their bodies as they trekked forward.

Most people are drinking within limits of normality, but every now and then, I see a case where a client will be using the philosophy that the more they take in, the better their health. Nothing could be further from the truth!

The body will be in full flush mode continually when people start to drink much more than they need. Kidneys in overload will start to push lots of fluid out, taking away vital electrolytes and minerals with it. Once our mineral reserves are down, so are our defences. Loss of immunity will be the first sign of this illness, with heart rate problems to follow if it progresses.

By all means, drink small amounts often, but if you find yourself making endless trips to the bathroom, maybe you need to consider cutting back. Less trips to the bathroom means more time to do the things in life that really make a difference.

Hydration—Such a Fine Line!

One of the best things you can do to ensure that you perform at your best is to give your body the right level of hydration. Your hydration level has everything to do with your blood volume.

If you don't think blood volume is important, then think again. If your body detects even a 1 per cent drop in blood volume, your heart will ramp up its rate in order to maintain pressure. This means that your heart rate will be elevated even before you start your training session.

The right hydration depends on factors such as activity levels and heat, but more than two and a half litres for those that are moderately active could start to be an excess.

Small quantities often offer better benefit than bucketing down large quantities in one hit.

When you know better, you will do better!

Having Trouble Sleeping at Night?

Lots of us believe that lack of hydration and minerals are signalled by a cramp.

Sometimes the signs of electrolyte imbalances are more subtle than that. Insomnia can be one of the first sign that things are not in balance.

Do you notice your eye twitching every so often? It may also be a sign that your electrolytes are lower than they should.

Drinking large amounts of water, excess sweating, and nightly trips to the toilet can sometimes mean that we lose lots of necessary minerals from our bodies.

Try a week of the following: Taking an electrolyte drink twice daily for a week, along with small amounts of fluid at regular intervals. This simple strategy could just see you back on track to a good night's sleep. Drink well, sleep well then go like hell!

Closing Paragraph

Hopefully, you have found some of the tips in this book helpful in getting you to look at training, nutrition, and mindset through a different set of eyes.

Understanding what it takes with simple yet effective strategies can be the difference between success and failure when it comes to bettering one's health.

Achieving optimum health should be the most important thing in your life. Sometimes we don't realise the importance of our health until it is taken away from us. For optimum health, we need to make changes in more than just one area of our lives.

If this book can get you to make even a few changes for the better, then it will have been well worth the read. Taking some time out to read a few lines at the end of each day and making a few changes will see you living the life that you have never thought possible.

Your health is your wealth, so go out, and grab it with both hands. Your body will thank you for it!

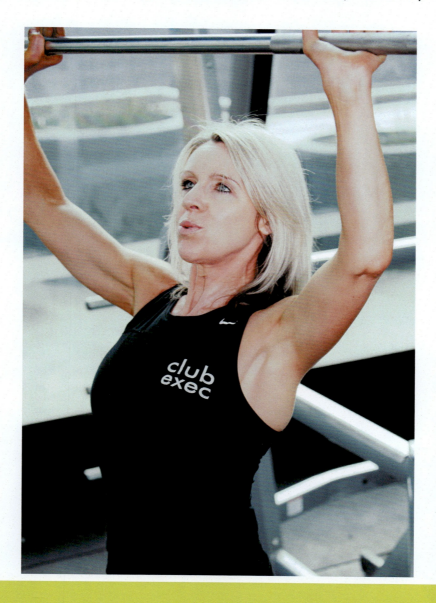

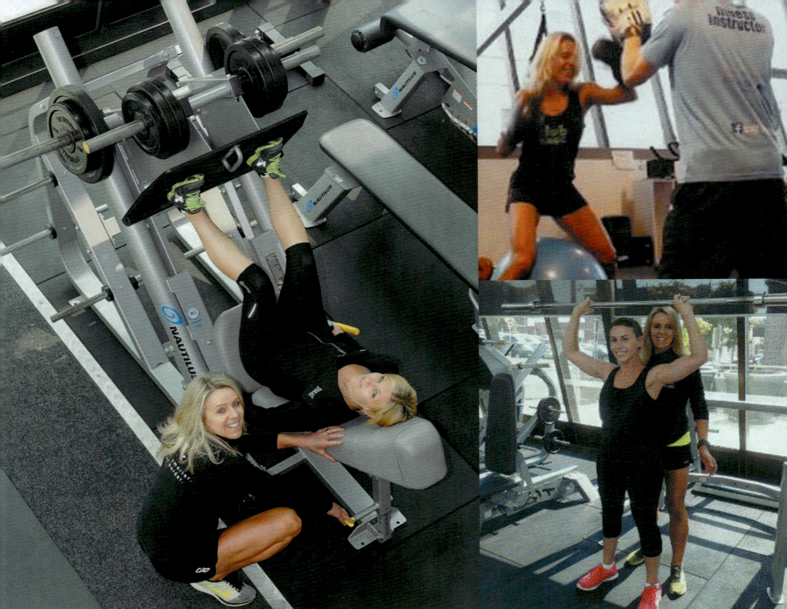

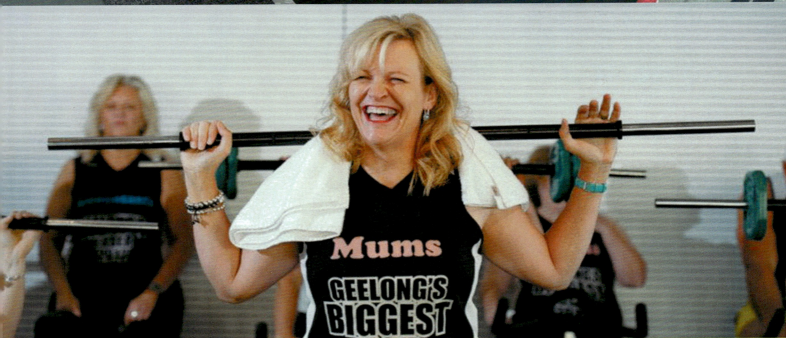

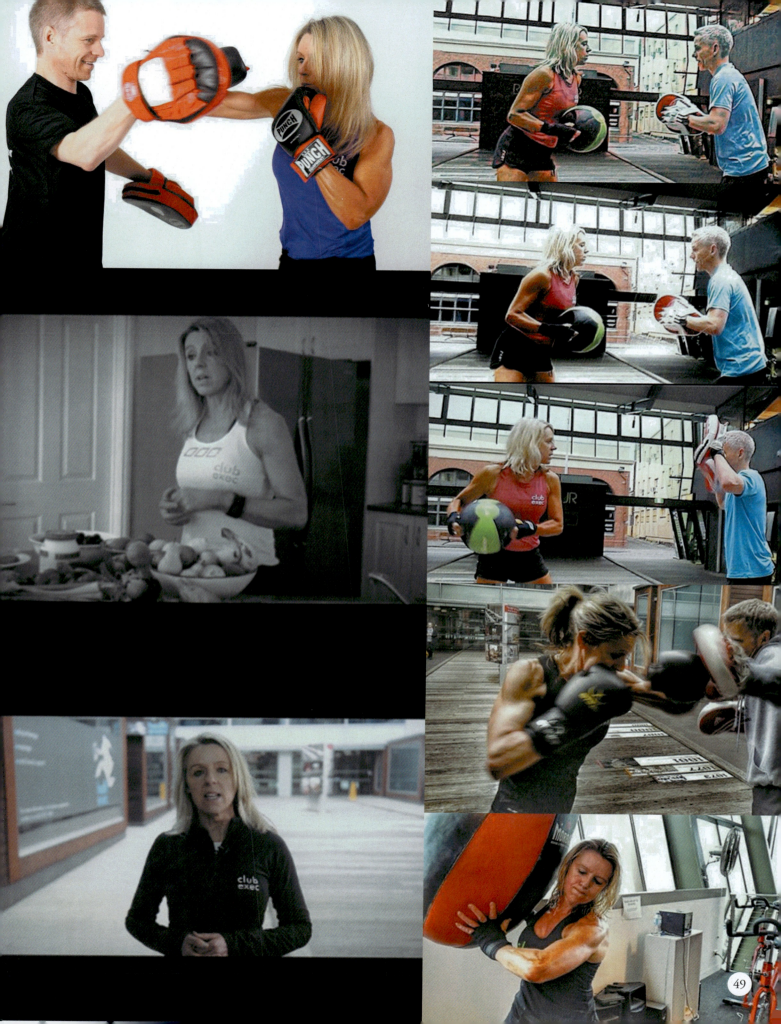

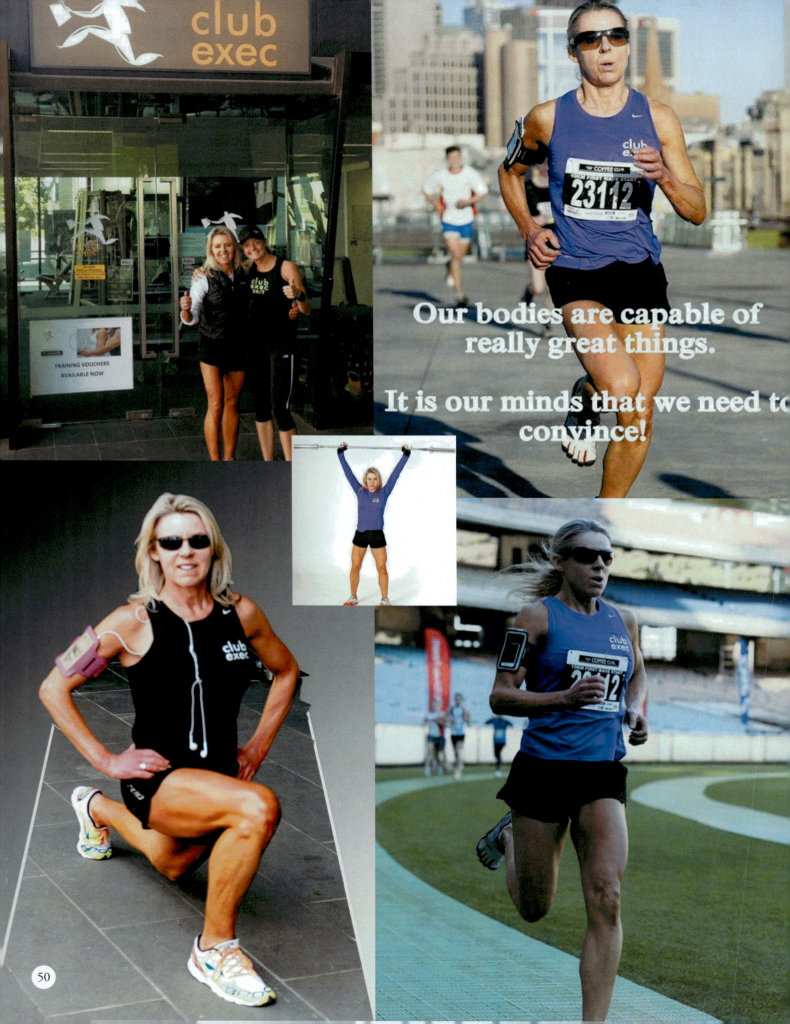

Our bodies are capable of really great things.

It is our minds that we need to convince!

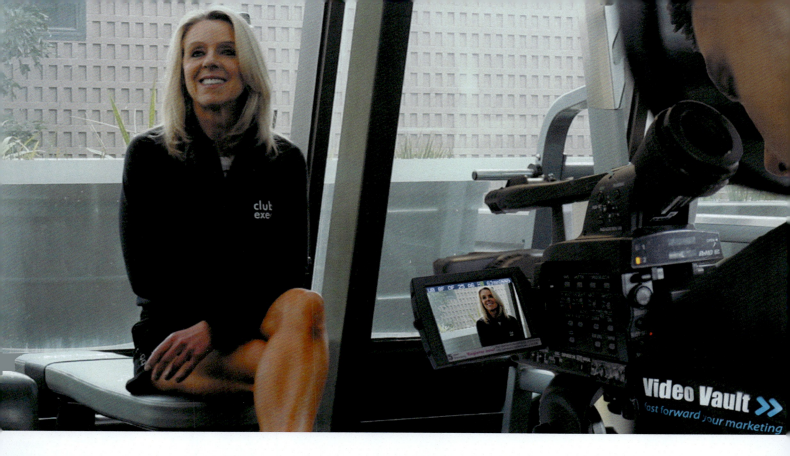

About the Author

Robyn Reimers is the managing director and founder of Club Exec Health Club, which is located on the corner of Clare and Corio streets in Central Geelong, Victoria, Australia. The club's motto is 'Train smarter, not harder' with a focus on providing a high level of service and a strong commitment to client care.

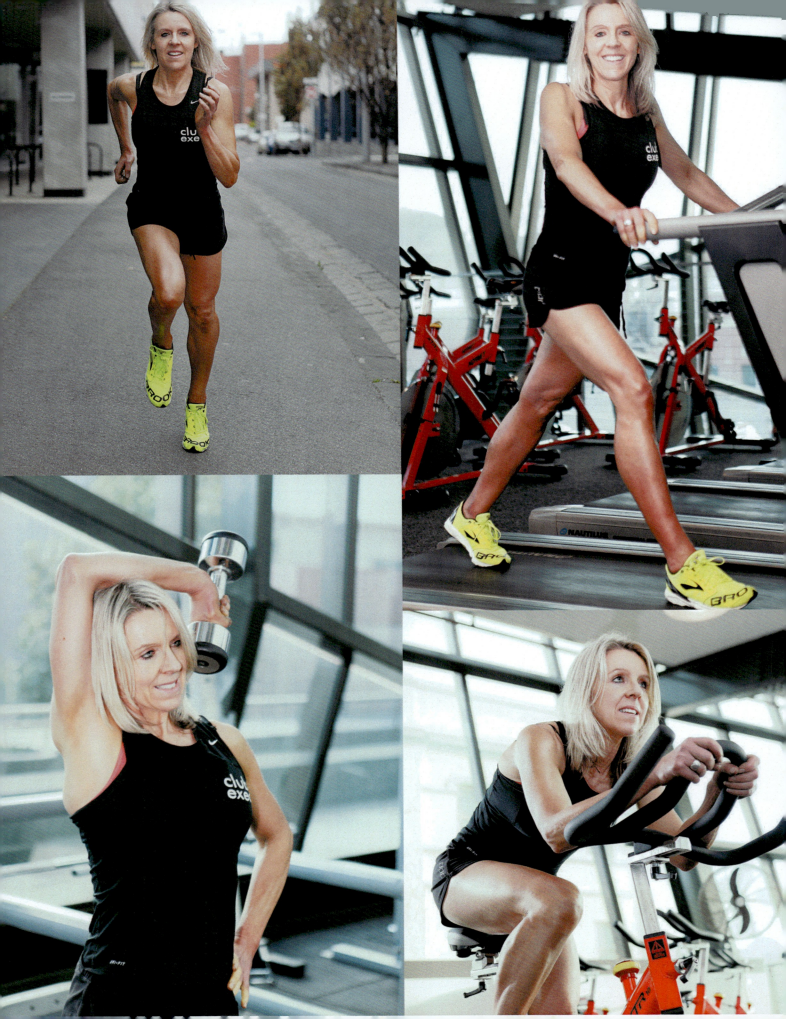